ULTIMATE CHAIR YOGA FOR SENIORS OVER 60

Simple and Gentle Exercises to Improve Flexibility, Strength, and Balance in Just 15 Minutes a Day

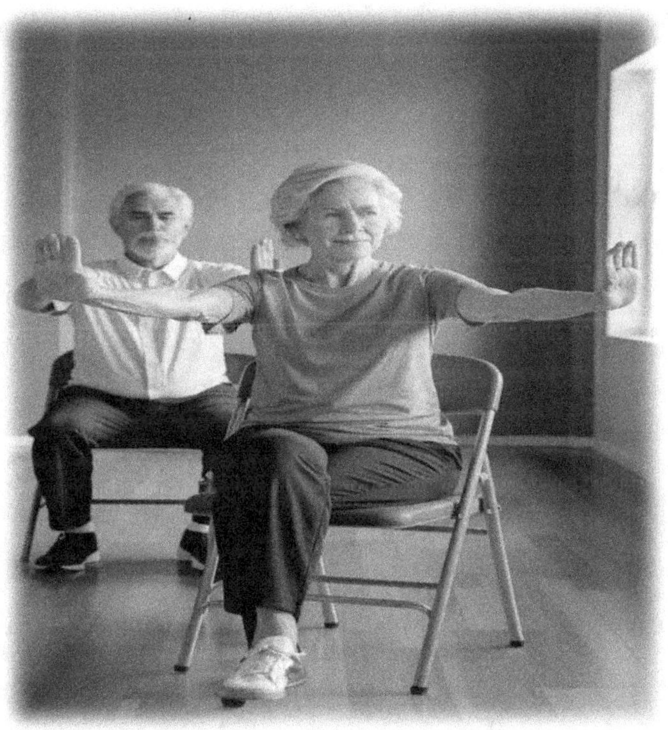

HARRY LAVELLE

TABLE OF CONTENT

INTRODUCTION

Meet John and Mary, a couple in their early seventies, who had always enjoyed an active lifestyle. However, as the years went by, they began to notice a creeping sense of lethargy. Their once-vibrant days were now spent mostly sitting, watching TV, and reminiscing about their more energetic years. The problem was clear: they were losing their vitality and zest for life.

John felt the weight of his own body every time he got up from his chair, and Mary's joints ached with even the smallest of movements. They were stuck in a cycle of inactivity, fearing that their age was finally catching up to them. But deep down, they refused to believe that this was the life they were destined to live.

Then, one afternoon, while browsing online for ways to regain their lost energy, they stumbled upon a book titled

"Ultimate Chair Yoga for Seniors Over 60." Intrigued, they decided to give it a try. The promise of regaining strength and flexibility, all from the comfort of a chair, seemed almost too good to be true. But something about the approach spoke to them—it felt doable and safe.

This book is designed specifically for seniors like John and Mary, who want to improve their quality of life without risking injury. Chair yoga provides a gentle yet effective way to increase mobility, improve balance, and enhance overall well-being. It breaks down the barrier of traditional yoga practices, making them accessible for those who may have physical limitations.

As a certified yoga instructor with over 20 years of experience working with seniors, I've seen firsthand the transformative power of chair yoga. My methods have been refined over the years, focusing on the specific needs and challenges faced by older adults. This book is the culmination of those years of experience, filled with exercises that have helped countless seniors regain control of their bodies and lives.

John and Mary found themselves slowly coming back to life. Through chair yoga, they experienced a renewed sense of flexibility and strength. Their daily aches diminished, and their mood improved significantly. No longer did they feel trapped by their age or physical limitations. Instead, they embraced each day with a newfound enthusiasm.

The benefits of chair yoga are extensive:

- Improved flexibility and strength
- Enhanced balance and coordination
- Increased energy and vitality
- Reduced stress and anxiety
- Better posture and joint health

Within weeks, John and Mary felt like new people. They could walk longer distances without fatigue and enjoyed their hobbies with a vigor they hadn't felt in years. Their friends noticed the change, asking them what their secret was.

This book includes real-life testimonials from others who have embraced chair yoga and experienced similar transformations. It's not just theory—it's proven practice.

By following the program outlined in this book, you too can reclaim your vitality. You'll discover the joy of movement, improve your health, and find a renewed sense of purpose. It's a promise that, if followed, can lead to significant changes in your life.

The biggest mistake you can make is to delay taking action. Every day spent in inactivity is a day lost. This book offers a straightforward, easy-to-follow plan that requires no special equipment or previous experience. Don't wait until tomorrow to start living your best life today.

Spy into the pages ahead and discover how you can transform your life with chair yoga. Let John and Mary's journey inspire you to take the first step. Embrace the possibilities that await and join the growing community of seniors who refuse to let age define them.

Whether you're looking to improve your health, regain energy, or simply feel better each day, "Ultimate Chair Yoga for Seniors Over 60" is your guide to achieving those goals. Start your journey now and see the difference it can make in your life.

CHAPTER 1

UNDERSTANDING CHAIR YOGA

What is Chair Yoga?

Chair yoga is an innovative approach to traditional yoga designed to make the practice more accessible, especially for seniors or individuals with mobility challenges. Unlike conventional yoga, chair yoga uses a stable chair as a supportive tool, enabling participants to experience the benefits of yoga without the need for complex poses or floor exercises.

The Origins of Chair Yoga

Yoga has a rich history dating back thousands of years, rooted in ancient Indian philosophy. Chair yoga emerged as a modern adaptation, recognizing the need for inclusivity in the practice. It was developed to bridge the gap for those who might find traditional yoga intimidating or physically demanding.

Key Principles

Chair yoga retains the fundamental principles of traditional yoga: balance, flexibility, strength, and mindfulness. It emphasizes gentle movements that are easy on the joints, making it ideal for seniors or those with physical limitations. By incorporating breathing exercises and meditation, chair yoga provides a holistic approach to wellness, promoting mental and physical harmony.

Benefits of Chair Yoga

- ❖ **Improved Flexibility and Strength**
  - ➤ Chair yoga helps enhance flexibility and build muscle strength through gentle stretching and resistance exercises. This can lead to better posture, reduced risk of falls, and improved overall mobility.
- ❖ **Enhanced Mental Well-being**
  - ➤ The practice incorporates mindfulness and breathing techniques, reducing stress and promoting mental clarity. This focus on relaxation can lead to improved sleep and a more positive outlook on life.
- ❖ **Accessibility and Convenience**
  - ➤ Since chair yoga can be practiced anywhere with a chair, it offers unmatched convenience. This makes it easy to integrate into daily routines, whether at home or in a community setting.

Who Can Benefit?

Chair yoga is not just for seniors. It's suitable for anyone seeking a low-impact exercise routine, including those recovering from injuries, pregnant individuals, or those who sit for long periods. Its adaptability allows for customized sessions that meet individual needs and fitness levels.

Getting Started

To begin chair yoga, all you need is a sturdy chair without wheels and some comfortable clothing. Sessions can range from five to thirty minutes, making it easy to fit into even the busiest schedules. Whether you're looking to start your day with energy or wind down in the evening, chair yoga offers a flexible approach to integrating wellness into your life.

Chair yoga offers a transformative approach to maintaining health and well-being for seniors. As we age, staying active becomes crucial, yet traditional exercise methods can often feel daunting. Chair yoga provides a gentle, accessible way to experience the physical and mental benefits of yoga, tailored specifically for seniors.

Enhanced Mobility and Flexibility

One of the primary benefits of chair yoga is improved mobility. As we age, joints can become stiff, and movement may feel restricted. Chair yoga focuses on gentle stretches and poses that increase flexibility without straining the body. This increased range of motion can lead to better posture, greater ease in daily activities, and a reduced risk of injury.

Strength Building

Despite its gentle approach, chair yoga effectively builds muscle strength. By engaging various muscle groups through controlled movements, seniors can maintain and even enhance their strength. This is essential for supporting bone health and preventing the onset of osteoporosis, contributing to overall physical resilience.

Improved Balance and Coordination

Falls are a significant concern for seniors, often leading to severe injuries. Chair yoga helps improve balance and coordination through exercises that enhance body awareness and stability. By regularly practicing balance-focused poses, seniors can gain confidence in their movements, reducing the likelihood of falls.

Stress Reduction and Mental Clarity

Chair yoga incorporates mindfulness and deep breathing techniques that significantly reduce stress and anxiety. For seniors, this can mean a marked improvement in mental clarity and emotional well-being. The calming effects of yoga promote better sleep, enhance focus, and foster a sense of peace, making everyday challenges more manageable.

Social Connection and Community

Participating in chair yoga classes offers more than just physical benefits; it provides an opportunity for social interaction. Many seniors experience isolation, which can negatively impact mental health. Chair yoga classes foster a sense of community, allowing individuals to connect with others, share experiences, and build friendships, contributing to a happier and more fulfilling life.

Customizable and Adaptable

Chair yoga is incredibly adaptable, making it suitable for seniors with varying levels of fitness and mobility. Whether seated or using the chair for support, exercises can be modified to suit individual needs. This flexibility ensures that everyone can participate and benefit, regardless of their physical condition.

Pain Management

Chronic pain is a common issue among seniors, often affecting quality of life. Chair yoga offers a gentle way to alleviate pain through movement and stretching. By increasing circulation and promoting relaxation, it can help manage symptoms of arthritis, back pain, and other chronic conditions, leading to an improved sense of well-being.

Independence and Quality of Life

Perhaps the most significant benefit of chair yoga for seniors is the promotion of independence. By maintaining physical health, seniors can continue to perform daily tasks with ease, preserving their autonomy. This independence enhances self-esteem and quality of life, allowing seniors to enjoy their golden years to the fullest.

Chair yoga is a powerful tool for seniors seeking to maintain their health and vitality. By offering a safe, effective, and enjoyable form of exercise, it empowers individuals to take control of their well-being. Whether practiced alone or in a group, chair yoga is an invitation to embrace a healthier, more active lifestyle, unlocking the full potential of aging gracefully.

CHAPTER 2

PREPARING FOR PRACTICE

Setting Up a Safe Environment for Chair Yoga

Creating a safe environment for chair yoga is essential to ensure a positive and effective experience. Whether you're practicing at home or in a group setting, a secure space allows seniors to focus on their movements and breathe deeply without distraction or risk.

Choosing the Right Space

The first step in setting up a safe environment is selecting an appropriate location. Ideally, this should be a quiet, well-lit room with ample space to move around. Ensure that the flooring is stable and non-slip, reducing the risk of accidents. If practicing at home, consider using a space free from clutter, with a clear area around the chair to prevent any potential hazards.

Selecting the Right Chair

The choice of chair is crucial for a safe and effective practice. Look for a sturdy chair with a straight back and no arms, providing adequate support during poses. The chair should be stable and placed on a non-slip surface, such as a yoga mat, to prevent movement. Ensure the seat height allows the feet to rest flat on the floor, promoting proper alignment and stability.

Gathering Necessary Props

In addition to a suitable chair, having the right props can enhance comfort and accessibility. Consider using yoga blocks, straps, and cushions to modify poses and provide additional support. These props can be particularly helpful for individuals with limited mobility or flexibility, allowing them to achieve the benefits of each pose safely.

Ensuring Proper Ventilation

A well-ventilated space is essential for maintaining comfort during practice. Fresh air contributes to overall well-being and helps prevent overheating. If possible, open windows or use a fan to keep the air circulating. A comfortable room temperature will ensure participants feel relaxed and focused throughout the session.

Creating a Calm Atmosphere

The environment should be peaceful and free from distractions. Soft lighting, soothing music, or nature sounds can enhance relaxation and concentration. Consider incorporating elements like plants or calming artwork to create a tranquil atmosphere that promotes mindfulness and presence.

Safety Precautions and Considerations

Before starting, ensure that all participants are aware of their personal limits and any health considerations. Encourage seniors to listen to their bodies and avoid pushing beyond their comfort zone. It's essential to provide modifications and alternatives for each pose, allowing everyone to participate safely and comfortably.

Encouraging Mindful Practice

Mindfulness is a core aspect of chair yoga, promoting awareness of the body and breath. Encourage participants to focus on their breathing and to move slowly and deliberately. This mindful approach reduces the risk of injury and enhances the mental and emotional benefits of the practice.

Establishing Clear Instructions

Clear communication is key to a successful chair yoga session. Provide detailed instructions for each pose, emphasizing alignment and safety. Demonstrating the poses or using visual aids can help participants understand and follow along more easily.

Emergency Preparedness

While chair yoga is generally safe, it's important to be prepared for any unexpected situations. Keep a first aid kit nearby and ensure that participants know how to seek help if needed. Having a plan in place provides peace of mind and ensures that any issues can be addressed promptly and efficiently.

Necessary Equipment and Modifications

Starting with a chair yoga journey requires minimal equipment, making it accessible and convenient for seniors. The key is to ensure comfort and safety while maximizing the benefits of each session. Here's a detailed guide to the necessary equipment and modifications that can enhance your chair yoga practice.

Essential Equipment

❖ **Stable Chair:**
  ➢ A sturdy chair without wheels is crucial. It should have a straight back and no arms to allow freedom of movement. Ensure that the chair is positioned on a non-slip surface to prevent sliding.
❖ **Yoga Mat:**
  ➢ Placing a yoga mat under the chair can provide additional stability. It offers grip for your feet during standing poses or transitions.
❖ **Supportive Cushions:**
  ➢ Cushions or folded blankets can be used to elevate the seat or provide lumbar support. This is especially useful for individuals with lower back issues.
❖ **Yoga Blocks:**

> Blocks can aid in reaching the floor or providing support during certain stretches. They offer stability and help maintain proper alignment.

❖ **Straps or Belts:**
> Yoga straps or even a sturdy belt can assist in deepening stretches. They're useful for those with limited flexibility.

❖ **Resistance Bands:**
> These can add a gentle challenge to your practice, helping to build strength gradually. They're excellent for arm and leg exercises.

Modifications for Safety and Comfort

Chair yoga is adaptable, making it ideal for seniors with varying levels of mobility. Here are some modifications to consider:

❖ **Range of Motion:**
> Encourage gentle movements. Avoid pushing into discomfort or pain. Each pose can be modified to accommodate personal limitations.

❖ **Seated Variations:**
> Many traditional yoga poses can be adapted to a seated position. This reduces the risk of falls and allows for a focus on balance and control.

❖ **Breathing Techniques:**
> Emphasize deep, mindful breathing. This can enhance relaxation and concentration. Breath

awareness is vital, especially during challenging poses.

❖ **Pacing:**
- ➢ Allow time between poses for rest and reflection. Slow transitions reduce strain and allow for mindful practice.

❖ **Use of Props:**
- ➢ Props can assist with balance and provide confidence in performing poses. They help maintain alignment and prevent injury.

❖ **Instructor Guidance:**
- ➢ Consider sessions with a qualified instructor, especially when starting out. They can offer personalized modifications and ensure correct technique.

Creating a Comfortable Space

Ensure your practice area is inviting and free of distractions. Good lighting, fresh air, and soothing music can enhance the experience. Having water nearby is important to stay hydrated.

CHAPTER 3

25

FUNDAMENTAL POSES

Detailed Instructions for Beginners

Starting on a chair yoga journey can be a transformative experience, especially for seniors. This practice offers a gentle yet effective way to enhance physical health and mental well-being. Here, we provide step-by-step instructions to help you start your chair yoga practice with confidence and ease.

Getting Started: The Basics

Before diving into the exercises, ensure you have a comfortable, stable chair and a quiet space. Wear loose, breathable clothing to allow for free movement. Keep a water bottle nearby to stay hydrated.

Warm-Up: Preparing Your Body

❖ **Seated Breathing:**

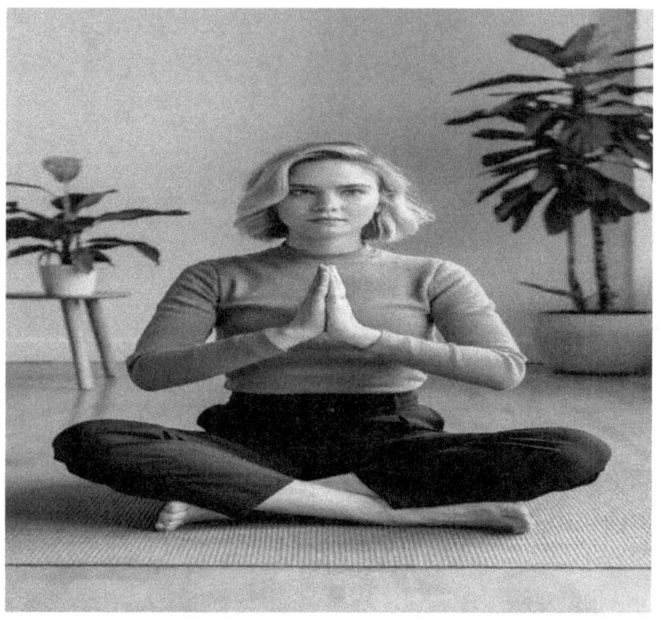

> Sit comfortably with your feet flat on the ground. Close your eyes and take a few deep breaths, inhaling through your nose and exhaling through your mouth. Focus on the rhythm of your breath, calming your mind and preparing your body for movement.

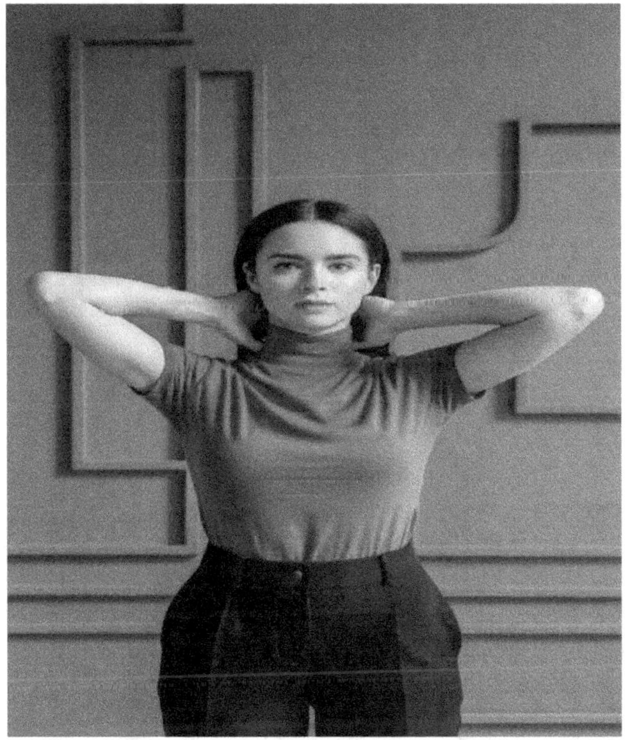

➤ Gently tilt your head forward and slowly roll it in a circle. Do this a few times in one direction, then switch. This releases tension in the neck and shoulders.

❖ **Shoulder Shrugs:**

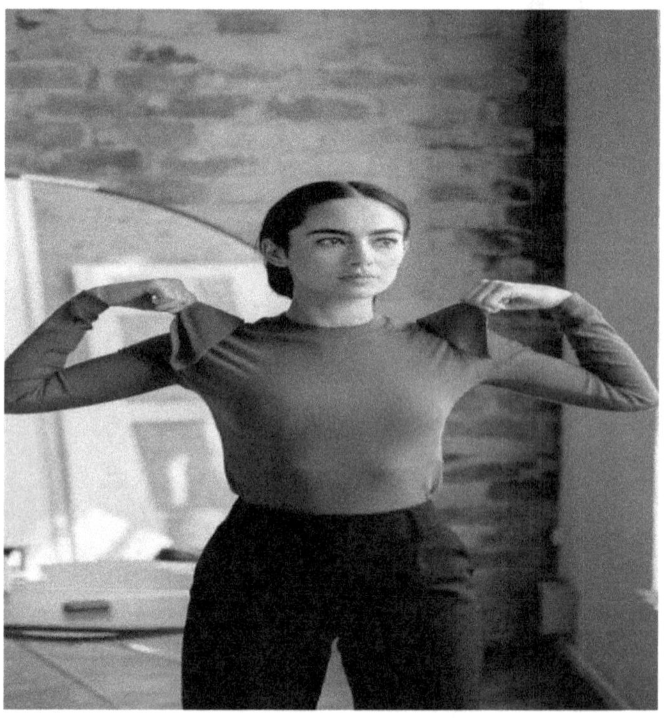

➢ Raise your shoulders towards your ears and then release them back down. Repeat several times to loosen tight muscles.

Core Exercises: Building Strength and Flexibility

❖ **Seated Forward Bend:**

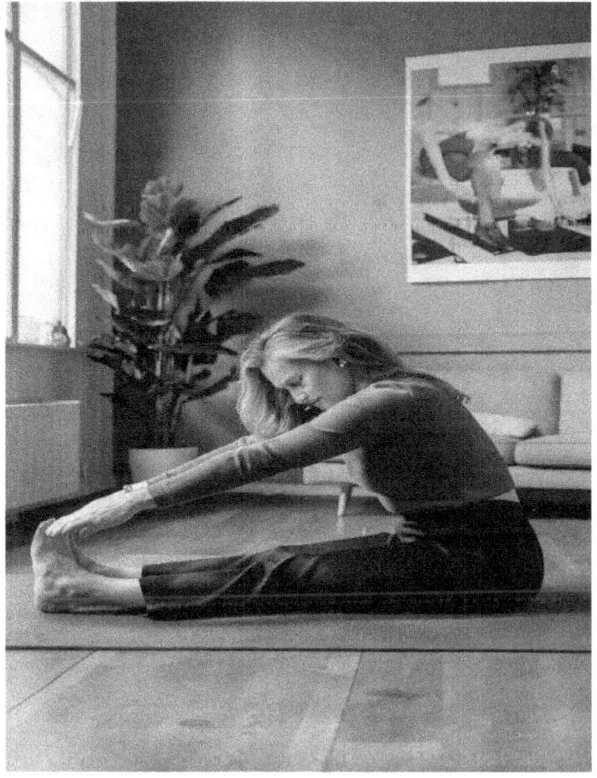

Sit at the edge of your chair with feet hip-width apart. Inhale, lengthening your spine, and exhale as you hinge forward from the hips, reaching towards the floor. This stretches the back and hamstrings.

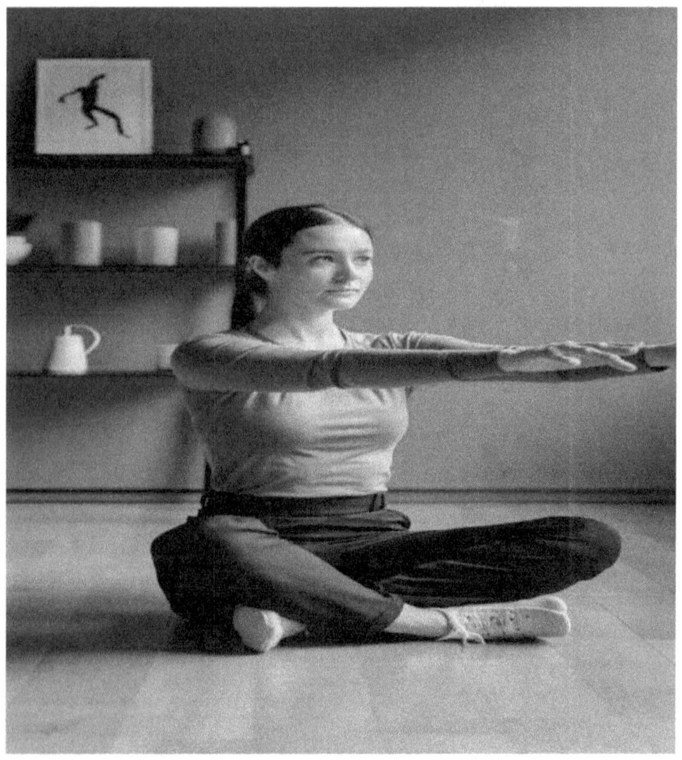

> ➢ Place your hands on your knees. Inhale, arching your back and lifting your chest (Cow Pose). Exhale, rounding your spine and tucking your chin (Cat Pose). Repeat several times to increase spinal flexibility.

❖ **Seated Twist:**

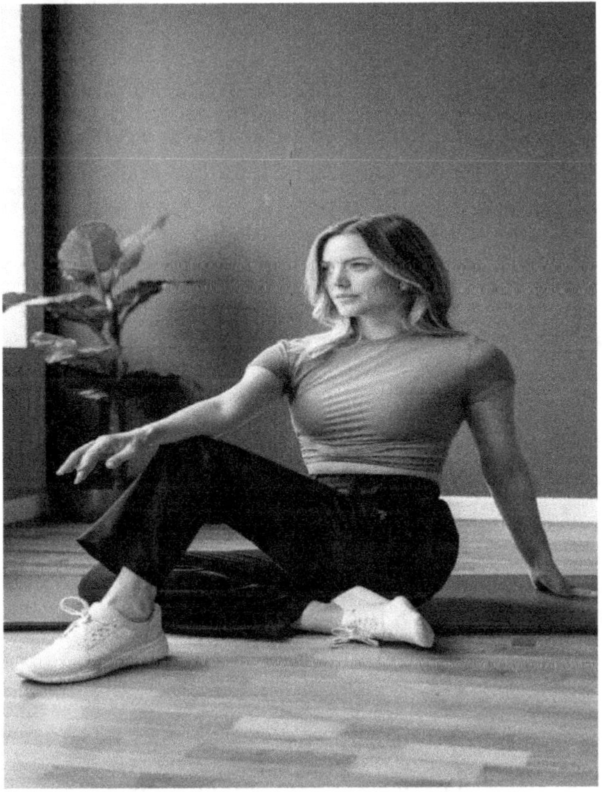

➢ Sit upright with feet flat. Inhale, then on the exhale, gently twists to the right, placing your left hand on the outside of your right knee. Hold for a few breaths, and then switch sides. This improves spinal mobility and digestion.

Balance and Coordination

- ❖ **Seated Leg Lifts:**
    - ➢ Sit with your back straight. Extend one leg out in front, keeping it straight. Hold for a few seconds, then lower. Alternate legs to strengthen the thighs and improve balance.
- ❖ **Ankle Circles:**
    - ➢ Extend one leg and rotate your foot in circles. This enhances ankle flexibility and prevents stiffness.

Relaxation and Cool Down

- ❖ **Seated Side Stretch:**
    - ➢ Raise your right arm overhead and lean to the left, stretching your side. Hold and breathe, then switch sides. This lengthens the torso and improves flexibility.
- ❖ **Guided Relaxation:**
    - ➢ Sit back comfortably, close your eyes, and take deep breaths. Imagine a peaceful place, allowing your body to relax completely. This helps in reducing stress and anxiety.

Building Confidence and Consistency

Starting with short, manageable sessions is key. Aim for 10 to 15 minutes a day, gradually increasing as you become more comfortable. Consistency is crucial; regular practice will lead to noticeable improvements in flexibility, strength, and overall well-being.

Tips for Success

- **Listen to Your Body:** Never push into pain. Modify poses as needed, using props like blocks or straps for support.
- **Stay Present:** Focus on your breath and movements. Mindfulness enhances the benefits of each pose.
- **Celebrate Progress:** Acknowledge your achievements, no matter how small. Each step forward is a victory.

CHAPTER 4

DEVELOPING A ROUTINE

Customizing your practice

Creating a personalized yoga practice is essential for seniors to address individual needs and enhance their well-being. Here's how to customize your chair yoga routine

Understanding Your Needs

Every person has unique health conditions, flexibility levels, and fitness goals. Begin by assessing your own physical abilities and any limitations. Are there specific areas you wish to focus on, such as improving balance or relieving joint pain? Knowing your needs helps tailor a practice that is both effective and safe.

Adapting Poses

Chair yoga offers various poses that can be modified to suit your comfort level. For example, if you have tight hips, focus on gentle hip openers that can be performed while seated. Use props like cushions or yoga blocks to provide additional support. Experiment with different variations of a pose to find what feels right for your body.

Creating a Routine

Structure your practice by choosing a mix of poses that address your goals. Begin with a warm-up to gently stretch and prepare your muscles. Include core exercises to enhance stability and balance. Conclude with a relaxing cool-down to help your body unwind and recover. A well-rounded routine ensures that all aspects of your fitness are addressed.

Listening to Your Body

Pay attention to how your body responds to each pose. It's crucial to listen to your body's signals and adjust accordingly. If a movement causes discomfort or pain, modify the pose or skip it entirely. Consistency and patience are key; progress at your own pace to avoid injury.

Incorporating Breathing Techniques

Breathing plays a significant role in yoga practice. Incorporate deep breathing exercises to promote relaxation and mindfulness. Practicing conscious breathing can help manage stress and improve concentration, making your yoga sessions more effective.

Setting Goals

Define clear, achievable goals for your yoga journey. Whether it's increasing flexibility, building strength, or enhancing mental clarity, setting goals keeps you motivated. Track your progress and celebrate milestones to maintain enthusiasm and commitment.

Utilizing Resources

Consider using online videos, books, or classes specifically designed for seniors to guide your practice. These resources can provide new ideas and ensure you're performing poses correctly. If possible, consult with a certified yoga instructor who can offer personalized advice and adjustments.

Staying Consistent

Consistency is vital for reaping the benefits of yoga. Aim to practice regularly, whether it's daily or a few times a week. Establishing a routine helps reinforce the habit and leads to gradual improvements over time.

Embracing Flexibility

Remember, yoga is not just about physical flexibility but also about adapting to change. Be open to altering your routine as your needs and abilities evolve. This adaptability allows your practice to grow with you, ensuring it remains beneficial and enjoyable.

By customizing your chair yoga practice, you create a personalized path to wellness that suits your lifestyle and health goals. Enjoy the journey of self-discovery and improved well-being as you embrace this accessible form of exercise.

Tips for Consistency and Progress for ultimate

Staying consistent with your chair yoga practice can lead to remarkable progress in flexibility, strength, and overall well-being. Here are some tips to help you maintain regular practice and see continuous improvement:

Set Clear Goals

Begin by defining what you want to achieve with your chair yoga practice. Whether it's enhancing flexibility, improving balance, or reducing stress, having clear goals provides direction and motivation. Write these goals down and revisit them regularly to track your progress.

Create a Schedule

Establish a routine by setting aside specific times for your practice. Consistency is key, so choose times that fit seamlessly into your daily life. Whether it's morning, afternoon, or evening, find a time when you feel most energized and focused.

Start Small

If you're new to chair yoga, start with short, manageable sessions. Even five to ten minutes a day can be beneficial. As you become more comfortable, gradually increase the duration of your practice. This approach prevents burnout and helps build a sustainable habit.

Make It Enjoyable

Incorporate elements that make your practice enjoyable. Play calming music, use aromatherapy, or practice in a space that feels peaceful and inspiring. When you enjoy the process, you're more likely to stick with it.

Track Your Progress

Keep a journal to document your experiences and progress. Note any improvements in flexibility, strength, or mental clarity. Celebrate small victories to keep your motivation high. Tracking progress not only highlights your achievements but also identifies areas for further growth.

Find a Community

Join a local chair yoga class or an online community for seniors. Engaging with others who share similar goals can provide support and encouragement. Sharing experiences and learning from others can enrich your practice and make it more enjoyable.

Stay Mindful

Practice mindfulness by focusing on the present moment during your sessions. Concentrate on your breath, the movement of your body, and the sensations you feel. Mindfulness enhances the benefits of yoga by promoting relaxation and reducing stress.

Listen to Your Body

Pay attention to how your body feels before, during, and after practice. If you experience discomfort, modify the pose or take a break. Progress at your own pace and avoid comparing yourself to others. Your practice is unique to you.

Be Patient

Remember that progress takes time. Celebrate each milestone, no matter how small. Patience is essential; consistent practice will lead to gradual and lasting improvements.

Adapt as Needed

As you progress, adapt your routine to meet your evolving needs and goals. Incorporate new poses and challenges to keep your practice fresh and engaging. Flexibility in your approach allows you to continue growing and enjoying your practice.

Reward Yourself

Set up a reward system for maintaining consistency. Treat yourself to something special when you reach certain milestones. Rewards can provide additional motivation to stay on track.

By incorporating these tips into your chair yoga routine, you can create a sustainable practice that enhances your physical and mental well-being. Embrace the journey and enjoy the transformation that comes with regular practice.

CHAPTER 5

ENHANCING FLEXIBILITY AND STRENGTH

Targeted Exercises for Key Muscle Groups

In the quest for optimal fitness, understanding how to effectively target key muscle groups is crucial. Whether you're a seasoned athlete or a fitness newbie, incorporating targeted exercises can lead to significant improvements in strength, mobility, and overall well-being. Let's dive into the essentials of crafting a well-rounded workout routine that focuses on these vital areas.

Core Muscles: The Foundation of Stability

The core is the powerhouse of the body, providing stability and support for virtually every movement. To engage these muscles, exercises like planks and Russian twists are indispensable.

Planks not only strengthen the abdominal muscles but also engage the back, hips, and shoulders. Begin by holding a plank position for 30 seconds, gradually increasing the duration as your strength improves. For variety, try side planks to focus on the oblique muscles, adding a rotational movement to enhance the challenge.

Russian twists are excellent for working the obliques and improving rotational strength. Sit on the ground with your knees bent, lean back slightly, and twist your torso from side to side while holding a weight. This movement not only fortifies the core but also boosts balance and coordination.

Upper Body: Building Strength and Definition

Targeting the upper body involves exercises that enhance the chest, back, and arms. **Push-ups** are a classic choice, offering a comprehensive workout for the chest, triceps, and shoulders. Start with standard push-ups, then explore variations like diamond push-ups or incline push-ups to shift the focus and increase intensity.

Pull-ups are another staple for upper body strength, particularly for the back and biceps. If traditional pull-ups are challenging, consider using resistance bands for assistance. This modification allows you to build strength progressively while maintaining proper form.

For a focused arm workout, **tricep dips** are invaluable. Use a bench or chair, lower your body by bending your elbows, and then push back up. This movement effectively isolates the triceps, promoting muscle growth and endurance.

Lower Body: Power and Endurance

The lower body consists of powerful muscle groups that propel us through everyday activities. Exercises like squats and lunges are key for targeting the legs and glutes.

Squats are fundamental for building strength in the quads, hamstrings, and glutes. Keep your feet shoulder-width apart, lower your body as if sitting back into a chair, and ensure your knees don't extend past your toes. To increase difficulty, add weights or try single-leg squats for greater intensity.

Lunges are excellent for improving balance and coordination while strengthening the legs. Step forward with one leg, lower your hips until both knees are bent at a 90-degree angle, and push back to the starting position.

Variations such as reverse lunges or walking lunges can add variety and challenge to your routine.

Integrating Targeted Exercises

To maximize results, incorporate these targeted exercises into a balanced workout plan. Consider a mix of strength training and cardio to support muscle growth and cardiovascular health. Rest and recovery are equally important, allowing muscles to repair and grow stronger.

Remember, consistency is key. Gradually increase the intensity of your workouts and listen to your body to prevent injury. By focusing on targeted exercises, you not only build a stronger, more resilient body but also enhance your overall quality of life.

With dedication and the right approach, you'll find yourself achieving fitness goals you once thought were out of reach. Start today and experience the transformative power of targeted exercises.

Mastering Balance and Coordination: Techniques for Enhanced Stability and Grace

In a world where physical prowess and agility are prized, mastering balance and coordination can elevate both everyday activities and specialized performances. Whether you're aiming to enhance your athleticism or simply seeking to improve daily function, a variety of techniques can help you develop these essential skills. Let's explore some dynamic strategies to sharpen your balance and coordination, leading to a more harmonious and controlled movement experience.

The Foundation: Understanding Balance and Coordination

Balance refers to the ability to maintain your center of gravity over your base of support, while coordination involves the smooth execution of movements. Together, they contribute to a fluid and efficient physical performance. To improve these abilities, it's crucial to engage in exercises that challenge and enhance both.

Techniques for Enhancing Balance

1. Single-Leg Stands: This classic exercise is fundamental for building balance. Begin by standing on one leg while keeping your core engaged. To increase difficulty, try closing your eyes or performing gentle leg lifts. This practice challenges your proprioception—the sense of where your body is in space—and strengthens the stabilizing muscles in your legs and core.

2. Balance Board Training: Using a balance board or wobble board introduces an element of instability that forces your body to engage and strengthen stabilizing muscles. Start with basic movements like shifting your weight from side to side or front to back. As you gain confidence, try more advanced techniques, such as squats or single-leg stands on the board, to further enhance your balance.

3. Tai Chi and Yoga: Both Tai Chi and yoga are excellent for improving balance through their focus on slow, deliberate movements and deep breathing. Tai Chi's flowing sequences encourage stability and control, while yoga poses like Tree Pose or Warrior III challenge and improve your balance. Integrating these practices into your routine can offer both mental and physical benefits.

Techniques for Boosting Coordination

1. Agility Drills: Agility drills, such as ladder drills or cone exercises, are great for refining coordination. These drills involve quick, precise movements that enhance your ability to control and direct your body. Practice running through an agility ladder with various foot patterns or weaving through cones to improve your reaction time and spatial awareness.

2. Hand-Eye Coordination Exercises: Activities that require hand-eye coordination, such as catching and throwing a ball or juggling, help fine-tune your reflexes and coordination. Start with simpler tasks like tossing a ball against a wall and catching it, then progress to more complex movements like juggling multiple objects to further challenge your skills.

3. Dance and Rhythmic Movement: Dancing is a fun and effective way to improve coordination. The rhythmic nature of dance movements and patterns enhances your ability to synchronize body movements and maintain timing. Join a dance class or follow online tutorials that focus on various styles, from salsa to hip-hop, to engage both your mind and body in a rhythmic dance routine.

Practical Integration: Daily Balance and Coordination

Incorporating balance and coordination techniques into your daily routine can yield remarkable improvements. Consider simple practices such as walking on uneven surfaces or performing balance exercises during TV commercials. Engaging in activities that challenge your balance and coordination regularly will help you build and maintain these vital skills.

By dedicating time to balance and coordination training, you'll not only enhance your physical performance but also enjoy greater ease in everyday activities. These techniques foster a deeper connection between your body and mind, promoting overall stability and fluidity. Embrace the journey towards mastering balance and coordination, and experience the profound benefits of a more stable and graceful life.

CHAPTER 6

BREATHING AND MINDFULNESS

Techniques to Enhance Relaxation: Cultivating a Calm and Centered Mind

In today's fast-paced world, finding moments of calm and relaxation can seem like a luxury. Yet, cultivating relaxation is essential for maintaining overall well-being and mental clarity. By adopting various relaxation techniques, you can transform stress and tension into tranquility and peace. Let's explore several effective methods to enhance relaxation, each offering unique benefits and practices to fit your lifestyle.

The Art of Mindful Breathing

Mindful breathing is a cornerstone of relaxation, focusing on the breath to anchor your mind and soothe your nervous system. To practice mindful breathing, find a quiet space where you can sit comfortably. Close your eyes and take slow, deep breaths in through your nose, allowing your abdomen to expand fully. Exhale gently through your mouth, letting go of any tension. This simple yet powerful practice calms the mind and body, reduces stress, and improves focus.

4-7-8 Breathing is another effective technique. Inhale through your nose for a count of four, hold your breath for a count of seven, and then exhale slowly for a count of eight. This pattern activates the parasympathetic nervous system, promoting relaxation and reducing anxiety. Repeat this cycle for several minutes, and you'll find yourself in a more serene state.

Progressive Muscle Relaxation

Progressive Muscle Relaxation (PMR) involves systematically tensing and then relaxing different muscle groups to release physical tension. Begin with your toes and work your way up to your head. Tense each muscle group for about five seconds, then release and focus on the sensation of relaxation that follows. This technique helps you become more aware of physical tension and promotes a deeper sense of relaxation throughout your body.

Visualization and Guided Imagery

Visualization and **guided imagery** are powerful tools for inducing relaxation through mental imagery. Find a comfortable position and close your eyes. Picture a serene and peaceful setting, such as a beach or a quiet forest. Engage all your senses by imagining the sounds, smells, and sensations of this tranquil place. Guided imagery often involves a narrator or recording leading you through calming scenarios, enhancing the effectiveness of the practice. By immersing yourself in these mental landscapes, you can escape the pressures of daily life and experience profound relaxation.

Gentle Movement Practices

Gentle movement practices, such as yoga and Tai Chi, are excellent for enhancing relaxation through mindful movement. Yoga combines breathing exercises with physical postures, promoting flexibility, strength, and relaxation. Poses like Child's Pose, Legs-Up-The-Wall, and Savasana are particularly effective for calming the mind and releasing tension.

Tai Chi, known for its slow, deliberate movements, is another practice that enhances relaxation. This ancient Chinese martial art focuses on the flow of energy through the body, fostering a sense of calm and balance. Practicing Tai Chi helps synchronize breath with movement, promoting a meditative state and reducing stress.

Aromatherapy and Sensory Techniques

Aromatherapy involves using essential oils to enhance relaxation. Scents like lavender, chamomile, and eucalyptus are known for their calming properties. You can diffuse these oils in your home, add a few drops to your bath, or apply them topically with a carrier oil. The soothing aromas can ease stress, improve sleep quality, and elevate your mood.

Sensory techniques, such as engaging in a warm bath or using soft, calming music, also contribute to relaxation. The sensory experience of warmth and gentle sounds creates a cocoon of comfort, helping to release accumulated stress and promote a serene state of mind.

Creating a Relaxation Routine

Integrating these relaxation techniques into your daily routine can significantly enhance your overall sense of well-being. Set aside specific times each day for relaxation practices, whether it's in the morning to start your day with calm or in the evening to unwind before bed. Consistency is key to reaping the long-term benefits of relaxation techniques.

By embracing these methods, you can cultivate a greater sense of peace and balance in your life. Whether through mindful breathing, muscle relaxation, mental imagery, gentle movement, or sensory indulgence, each technique offers a pathway to relaxation and stress relief. Prioritize these practices, and experience the transformative power of enhanced relaxation in every aspect of your life.

Integrating Mindfulness into Practice: Cultivating Presence and Purpose

In a world brimming with distractions and constant movement, mindfulness emerges as a beacon of clarity and calm. Integrating mindfulness into your daily practice can profoundly transform how you engage with your environment, enhancing focus, reducing stress, and fostering a deeper connection with yourself and others. Let's explore how to seamlessly weave mindfulness into your routine and harness its full potential for a more balanced and purposeful life.

Understanding Mindfulness

At its core, **mindfulness** is the practice of being fully present in the moment, without judgment. It involves paying deliberate attention to your thoughts, feelings, and surroundings, accepting them as they are. This heightened awareness helps you respond to situations with greater clarity and calm, rather than reacting impulsively.

Mindful Moments in Daily Routine

1. Mindful Mornings: Start your day with intention. Instead of rushing through your morning routine, take a few moments to center yourself. Begin with a mindful stretch or gentle yoga poses, focusing on your breath and bodily sensations. As you shower or prepare breakfast, pay attention to the sensory experiences—the warmth of the water, the aroma of your coffee. This practice sets a tone of awareness and presence for the rest of the day.

2. Mindful Eating: Transform your meals into opportunities for mindfulness. Instead of eating on autopilot, savor each bite with full attention. Notice the colors, textures, and flavors of your food. Chew slowly and appreciate the nourishment. This approach not only enhances your enjoyment of food but also improves digestion and helps prevent overeating.

3. Mindful Breathing: Throughout your day, take short breaks to focus on your breath. A few minutes of mindful breathing can ground you and reduce stress. Inhale deeply through your nose, allowing your abdomen to expand, then exhale slowly through your mouth. This simple practice can be done anywhere—at your desk, in the car, or during a walk—offering a moment of calm amidst your busy schedule.

Integrating Mindfulness into Work and Relationships

1. Mindful Work: Bring mindfulness to your professional life by incorporating focused work sessions. Set aside specific blocks of time for tasks, and during these periods, concentrate solely on the task at hand. Minimize distractions by turning off notifications and creating a clutter-free workspace. Practice single-tasking rather than multitasking to enhance productivity and maintain a sense of accomplishment.

2. Mindful Communication: Cultivate deeper connections with others through mindful communication. When engaging in conversations, listen actively and fully without interrupting. Pay attention to the speaker's words, tone, and body language. Respond thoughtfully rather than reactively, acknowledging the other person's perspective. This mindful approach fosters empathy, strengthens relationships, and reduces misunderstandings.

Incorporating Mindfulness Practices

1. Mindfulness Meditation: Dedicate a specific time each day to mindfulness meditation. Find a quiet space, sit comfortably, and focus on your breath or a guided meditation. Allow your thoughts to come and go without judgment, gently bringing your focus back to the present moment. Regular meditation practice helps build mental resilience and cultivates a deeper sense of inner peace.

2. Mindful Movement: Integrate mindfulness into physical activities like yoga, Tai Chi, or even walking. As you move, pay attention to your body's sensations, breath, and the rhythm of your movements. This mindful approach to exercise not only enhances physical benefits but also fosters a stronger mind-body connection.

Creating a Mindful Environment

1. Mindful Space: Designate a space in your home or office for mindfulness practice. This can be a corner with comfortable seating, calming decor, and minimal distractions. Use this space for meditation, reflection, or simply taking mindful breaks.

2. Mindful Technology Use: Approach technology with intention by setting boundaries and using apps designed to support mindfulness. Limit screen time, schedule regular digital detox periods, and utilize mindfulness apps for guided meditations or breathing exercises.

Embracing Mindfulness as a Lifestyle

Integrating mindfulness into practice is not a one-time effort but an ongoing journey. By incorporating these practices into your daily routine, work, and relationships, you cultivate a more mindful, present, and purposeful life. Embrace the art of mindfulness as a transformative tool for enhanced well-being, and experience the profound impact it can have on every facet of your existence.

CHAPTER 7

OVERCOMING CHALLENGES

Common Obstacles and Solutions

Chair yoga is an accessible and transformative practice for seniors, yet it can come with challenges. Understanding these obstacles and finding effective solutions is key to ensuring a rewarding experience. Here's how you can navigate common hurdles and continue your journey toward health and well-being.

1. Physical Limitations

Obstacle: Many seniors face physical limitations, such as joint pain, arthritis, or reduced flexibility, making some movements difficult.

Solution:

- **Modify Poses:** Use props like cushions or blocks to support the body. Modify poses to match your comfort level.

- **Listen to Your Body:** Encourage practicing mindfulness and awareness. If a pose causes pain, adjust it or skip it entirely.

2. Lack of Motivation

Obstacle: Staying motivated can be tough, especially when progress feels slow.

Solution:

- **Set Realistic Goals:** Break down your practice into achievable milestones. Celebrate small victories to maintain motivation.
- **Join a Community:** Connect with a local or online chair yoga group. Sharing experiences can inspire and encourage you to stay committed.

3. Fear of Injury

Obstacle: Concerns about falling or getting injured may deter some from trying new exercises.

Solution:

- **Focus on Safety:** Emphasize safety by practicing on a non-slip surface and using a sturdy chair.

- **Start Slow:** Begin with gentle, simple movements and gradually increase intensity as confidence grows.

4. Limited Space

Obstacle: Some seniors may feel constrained by small living spaces.

Solution:

- **Creative Arrangement:** Rearrange furniture to create a dedicated yoga area, even if it's just a corner of a room.
- **Minimal Equipment:** Highlight that chair yoga requires minimal equipment, making it adaptable to any environment.

5. Memory Challenges

Obstacle: Remembering sequences and poses can be challenging.

Solution:

- **Visual Aids:** Use charts or instructional videos for guidance. Visual aids can reinforce learning and aid recall.

- **Repetition and Routine:** Practice regularly to build familiarity with the sequences. Consistent repetition helps solidify memory.

6. Perception of Yoga

Obstacle: Some may view yoga as too difficult or not suitable for seniors.

Solution:

- **Educate and Inspire:** Share stories of other seniors who have successfully incorporated chair yoga into their lives.
- **Highlight Benefits:** Emphasize how chair yoga specifically addresses the needs of older adults, improving flexibility, balance, and overall wellness.

Starting on a chair yoga journey as a senior can be deeply rewarding. By understanding and addressing common obstacles, you can create a sustainable and enjoyable practice. Remember, yoga is a personal journey, and adapting it to suit your needs is perfectly acceptable.

Stay patient, listen to your body, and embrace the process. With perseverance and the right approach, chair yoga can become a cherished part of your daily routine, enhancing your quality of life in your golden years.

Adapting Poses for Individual Needs

As we age, our bodies change, and what once seemed like simple movements can become challenging. This is where the beauty of chair yoga shines—it's adaptable, gentle, and can be modified to meet individual needs. By tailoring poses to suit personal limitations and capabilities, seniors over 60 can safely and effectively enjoy the benefits of yoga.

Understanding the Importance of Adaptation

Chair yoga offers a unique opportunity to engage in a physical practice without the need for getting up and down from the floor. Adapting poses ensures that every individual, regardless of their physical condition, can participate and benefit. This inclusivity is crucial for maintaining a sense of community and encouraging consistent practice among seniors.

Key Principles of Adaptation

- ❖ **Listen to Your Body**
  - ➢ **Mindful Awareness:** Encourage seniors to tune into their bodies, recognizing any areas of tension or discomfort. Pain should never be ignored; it's a signal to modify or adjust the pose.
  - ➢ **Gentle Movements:** Start with slow, controlled movements to gauge how the body responds. Gradually increase the range of motion as comfort levels rise.
- ❖ **Use Props Effectively**
  - ➢ **Support and Stability:** Props such as cushions, yoga blocks, and straps can provide additional support and stability, making poses more accessible.
  - ➢ **Enhancing Comfort:** A rolled-up towel behind the lower back can support the lumbar spine, while placing a cushion on the seat can make prolonged sitting more comfortable.
- ❖ **Modify the Range of Motion**
  - ➢ **Partial Poses:** Instead of reaching for the toes, seniors can aim to touch their knees or shins, maintaining the benefits of the stretch without overexertion.

> **Adaptive Stretching:** Encourage participants to stretch only to the point of mild tension, avoiding any strain. Over time, flexibility will improve, allowing for deeper stretches.

Adapting Specific Poses

❖ **Seated Forward Bend**
  > **Modification:** Place a cushion on the thighs and fold forward, resting the forehead on the cushion. This reduces the strain on the lower back and hamstrings.
  > **Benefit:** Enhances flexibility in the spine and hamstrings while promoting relaxation.
❖ **Seated Spinal Twist**
  > **Modification:** Instead of a full twist, encourage a gentle turn, using the back of the chair for support. Avoid any forceful movements.
  > **Benefit:** Improves spinal mobility and aids in digestion, offering a gentle detoxifying effect.
❖ **Seated Warrior Pose**
  > **Modification:** Keep both feet firmly on the ground, extending the arms parallel to the floor. Adjust the depth of the lunge based on comfort.
  > **Benefit:** Strengthens the legs and core while enhancing balance and stability.

Personalizing the Practice

❖ **Assessing Individual Needs**

- ➢ **Initial Assessment:** Begin with a gentle assessment of each participant's abilities and limitations. This can include questions about previous injuries, current pain points, and overall fitness levels.
- ➢ **Ongoing Monitoring:** Regularly check in with participants to ensure the adaptations are still appropriate and make adjustments as needed.
- ❖ **Creating a Safe Environment**
  - ➢ **Sturdy Chairs:** Ensure chairs are stable and positioned on a non-slip surface to prevent accidents.
  - ➢ **Clear Instructions:** Provide clear, step-by-step instructions for each pose, emphasizing the importance of listening to the body and avoiding any discomfort.

Adapting poses for individual needs in chair yoga is not just about making the practice accessible; it's about honoring each person's unique journey. By customizing the practice, seniors can safely experience the physical, mental, and emotional benefits of yoga, fostering a sense of empowerment and well-being. Remember, the goal is progress, not perfection. Encourage patience, celebrate small victories, and enjoy the journey toward improved health and vitality.

With these adaptations, chair yoga becomes a powerful tool for seniors over 60, offering a pathway to enhanced flexibility, strength, and overall quality of life.

CONCLUSION

Imagine waking up each day with a renewed sense of energy and vitality. Picture the joy of moving with ease, free from the aches and stiffness that once held you back. This is not just a dream; it's the reality that many seniors have embraced through the transformative power of chair yoga.

As we age, maintaining physical activity becomes challenging. Many seniors face mobility issues, pain, and a lack of motivation, which can lead to a decline in overall well-being.

Chair yoga offers a gentle yet effective way to stay active. It's accessible to everyone, regardless of fitness level, and provides a holistic approach to health, addressing both the body and mind.

With years of experience in teaching yoga to seniors, I've witnessed firsthand the incredible changes this practice can bring. My expertise ensures that you are guided safely through each pose, with adaptations tailored to individual needs.

- **Improved Flexibility:** Gently stretching muscles increases your range of motion, making daily activities easier.
- **Enhanced Strength:** Regular practice builds muscle strength, supporting joints and preventing falls.
- **Better Balance:** Chair yoga improves stability, reducing the risk of injury.
- **Mental Clarity:** The mindfulness aspect of yoga enhances focus and reduces stress.

Consider Mary, a 72-year-old who struggled with chronic back pain. After incorporating chair yoga into her routine, she now enjoys pain-free days and more energy. Or John, who found his balance and coordination improved significantly, giving him the confidence to engage in activities he once avoided.

By committing to chair yoga, you're investing in your future health and happiness. This book provides the tools and guidance needed to transform your life, one gentle stretch at a time.

Every day spent inactive is a day lost to potential improvement. Don't wait for the perfect moment to start—begin your journey to better health now.

Dive into the pages of this book, follow the simple routines, and discover how chair yoga can enhance your life. Embrace the path to a more vibrant and active you.

Thank you for embarking on this journey with me. I hope "Ultimate Chair Yoga for Seniors Over 60" has inspired and empowered you. If you found value in this book, I'd be grateful if you could leave a 5-star review. Your feedback helps others discover the benefits of chair yoga and encourages them to take the first step toward a healthier lifestyle.

With gratitude and best wishes on your yoga journey.

9 798333 810489